The
Long
Farewell

Memories of Special Times

By

Marley West

First Published 2015

Typeset in Times New Roman
(14pt / 11pt)

Quick - Books

<u>DEDICATION</u>

Simply to my parents.

CONTENTS

<u>APPRECIATION</u>

*I would like to thank all who gave me so much inspiration
to complete this work. Writing this book rekindled so
many wonderful memories of family, friends and
characters and i thank you all for your support.
I thank my Mother. I thank my family.
Also my darling Wife.*

PREFACE

Suddenly my mobile phone began to vibrate, sounding out it's tune from the breast pocket of my shirt. Weary and half asleep i fumbled my shirt pocket, drawing it carefully so my tired eyes had time to focus on the screen spelling out the callers name.

'Hi Mom, how are you?' Rubbing the sleep from my eyes the voice so familiar to me came down the line, 'Hi Morris i am fine are you going to hospital today?', and trying not to sound surprised i answered, 'Yes later this evening. In fact i was going to ring you to see if you wanted me to come and pick you up?' I could hear the relief in Mom's voice as she replied, 'Oh please, will you!.

Mom was so independent, normally it would be me ringing her to offer my services and more often than not she would decline and i would arrive at the hospital to find her sat in the ward. Made her own way on the bus, however today was Sunday and the bus service was very hit and miss, to say the least. 'I don't want to be a burden' she would say when challenged on the subject. A burden, I thought, now that she will never be.

I found many women of Mom's age to be independent. I

put it down to the suffering and hardship they must of endured in the aftermath of the Second World War, being independent was a must i suppose, and i do know through reading reports and learning about local history that the area where my parents lived at the time of the war came under immense bombardment from the German Luftwaffe. Even though i found her independence to be irritating sometimes, i also found inspiration from it too.

Dad was asleep when we arrived, apparently he'd been awake most of the night before due to the pain.

'You know what i have noticed' Mom remarked straightening his bed sheets, 'The more he gets older, the more he looks like his Dad, your Grandad'.

It had been a long time since Grandad had passed away and as i sat looking at Dad, i began to think back.....

CHAPTER ONE

Sunday Morning Blues

The bright light of the early morning sun pierced like a knife, driving stronger and stronger into the back of my eye lids until finally, i was awake enough to turn my head away from the glare and open them and take a blurred look at the bed side clock. To which was announcing to the world in bright neon red figures it was 08.00am.

My head slumped back on my pillow disgusted at the sun and how it dare wake me at such a time on a Sunday morning, after all i was 15 years old, soon to be 16 years and was nearly a man. In my youthful world, Sundays were for laying in.

However this feeling of disgust soon passed as my nose caught the aroma drifting up from the kitchen below. It was bacon being cooked for breakfast and disgust soon turned into hunger as my stomach rumbled as if it was talking to me.

Jumping out of bed i headed for the bathroom, pulling up my underwear whilst itching my crotch along the way. I had only travelled half way when Dad suddenly darted from his bedroom holding a newspaper and hurried into the bathroom. That was the day when i came to realise my morning ritual, the one i thought private only to me was actually hereditary. However what worried me more was that i had glimpsed the future; People had always remarked how i was just like my Dad in looks and ways and to be honest the future looked bloody awful.

'Is that you i can hear Morris?', came Mom's voice from below. 'Yes Mom', i replied doing a Indian war dance across the landing, hoping it would stop my bladder from releasing as Mom sounded again, 'Don't you forget you promised to help your Grandad today with his garden'.

'Oh for god sake' i said out loud. Indeed i had forgot, it had totally slipped my mind, above all i had told him i would be there early and it was nearly 9am, and i was still dancing like Tonto waiting for the bathroom.

'He wont help you Morris' came Dads voice from behind the bathroom door. 'Dad please hurry up?' i asked frustrated, 'I really need the bathroom and i should be at Grandads now'.

Suddenly from the bathroom came a loud noise that echoed all around, as if someone had just broke wind whilst sat on a dustbin. 'Bloody hell Morris, i think i got

Louie Armstrong stuck up my arse' said Dad from within, 'What time was you suppose to clock on?' By this time Tonto had turned into Wayne Sleep, as due to desperation i was now doing cross legged squats like a ballet dancer. 'Early' i squeaked, i couldn't speak anymore, i was to busy concentrating on keeping my pee inside my bladder and not on the carpet, until CLICK and the bathroom door swung open, with Dad assuring me on his exit. 'Well that's the least of your worries lad, because your going to have to give that bathroom at least an hour to clear, bad glass of beer last night Son, Sorry and all that'. As I pushed passed Dad to finally get relief Mom's voice shouted up from the foot of the stairs 'Well you must have one every night!, i am fed up with that smell every morning, it's disgusting.', and as I stood with power washing the toilet basin with my urine, the horrid aroma within the bathroom drifted up my nose. Oh she does have a point, i thought.

'I think your in the dog house' i shouted knowing Dad could hear me in the next room.

'It looks like it' Dad replied in a huff 'And you can take that sarcasm from your voice my lad. This is what you've got to look forward to, it's called married life. I just hope she's done my grub?' I could still hear him mumbling as the floorboard creaked outside the bathroom door as he made his way to the top of the stairway.

I decided to abandon my normal morning routine of what i called the three S's, which was Shit, Shower and shave and just have number 1, which was a number two really if you get my meaning? I have often wondered why and how a toilet function came to be known as a number two, however i digress. Leaving the shower and shave until returning from helping Grandad, thinking this would be better, as i would probably need another after helping in Grandads garden. Also i could only hold my breath for so long in that horrid smell Dad left behind.

Mom was putting on her coat and head scarf as i came down the stairs, mumbling about how much weight she'd gained as she stood in front of the long dress mirror in the hall way. 'That will have to do' she said as she fingered her collar.

'You off out?' i asked reaching for my jacket.

'I'm off to see your Aunty Ethel' Mom replied opening the front door 'There is a breakfast in the oven make sure you have it before you go, oh and i hope you've put clean underwear on? Your not showing me up if anything happens, right i shall see you later'.

Clean underwear, where did that come from?, i ask myself. Mom was like that, she could come out with some silly statements. I remember once as a child, oh i must have been about seven and we were walking round a fruit and vegetable market. I must have been bored and started to misbehave, enough so that Mom in her wisdom told me 'If you carry on Morris i will get the man behind that stall to swap your head for a cabbage', i dreaded going to the market after that just in case they could.

It was up hill to Grandads house. I had set off running but running after a big breakfast took it's toll and i ended up walking after a short distance and as i turned the corner leading to his house, i could see his trouser bottom sticking up proud, as he worked his garden.

'Leave that Grandad!' i shouted 'I'm here now, i will do that.' Grandad looked up and with a blow of his cheeks, a rub of his back and a rye smile he complained, 'Eh i don't know lad, this garden seems to be getting harder and harder every year, do you think it might be my age Morris?. I think a cup of tea is in order don't you?, nip inside and tell Ma to put kettle on, that's a good lad.'

He always called Gran, .Ma for some reason. It sounded

funny and a bit weird to me because she was his Wife, however he never used her name Clara, it was always Ma, why i don't know?

Grandad Robert (Known as Bob) and Grandma Clara were my Grand parents from my Dads side of the family and even though i may sound biased, they were such a nice couple. Although very different in there ways and character. For example, my Grandma was a regular church goer, every Sunday morning or evening without fail. Her downfall, she was a worrier, she would worry and get stressed at the smallest thing. Yet Grandad? Well i think the only time i have seen him in church was at my eldest sisters wedding. He didn't have a care in the world. There could be a major trauma going on and he would be so relaxed about it, just letting everything go over his head.

'What you worrying for?' he would say to Grandma 'They can't hang you for it' or depending on the subject 'It will all come out in the wash.'

He could tell a story too. Many a time i had arrived to help him with a chore and instead spent the whole day listening to one of his stories. We would start what we was suppose to be doing then something would trigger his mind and he would always start the same way.

'I tell you what lad!' he would say, you knew after those words, a tale was going to be told. Now whether they were true or partly true but slightly exaggerated didn't matter, he could keep you fixated for hours. Stories of his childhood and the years before the First World War, stories of his life at sea after the war years. Although there was one period in his life that was never told or talked about, not with me anyway and that was during both wars.

You could tell when he'd reached that part, he would go quiet for a moment then after taking a puff on his tobacco pipe, he'd say. 'Think we'll leave it there for today Morris.'

It was mid-afternoon and glorious warm sunshine as i headed for home. I had left Grandad Bob contemplating whether it was to late in the year to plant some potatoes that he'd found going to seed and Grandma was in the kitchen making bread, even though you could buy it at the corner shop cheap enough. 'There's nothing like the taste of home made bread' she'd say when asked. She was right too.

As i walked home i couldn't help thinking whether Grandad was using these Sundays just to tell his stories as nothing got done again, apart from being on a dangerous trip into the North Sea on a fishing trawler. I didn't mind though.

It was on the way home i came across my friend Billy, his proper name was William but everyone called him Billy.

'Hay Mozzy' a voice shouted from behind. I turned to see a tall leggy frame in the distance, reminiscent of a stick insect on amphetamines running to catch up to me. Mozzy was a shortened street version of my name and like all nicknames over years it had stuck, although to be honest i preferred Mozzy. It was only my family that now called me Morris.

On his arrival, while trying to catch his breath, i could just make out what he was saying. 'I'm glad i have seen you mate, i have got your wallet, you left it behind last night.' I fumbled my inside jacket pocket, it was empty. 'Thanks Billy, i didn't even realise it was missing. Mind you mate i can't remember much about last night, can you?' Billy smiled and with a hint of sarcasm replied, 'I can remember winning Mozzy that's why it's empty.'

Billy was so lucky when it came to gambling. No matter whether it be cards, horses or dogs it was like he had the golden touch. Every Saturday night was spent at Billy's house playing cards for money, not much money of course as none of us had any. We played for pennies but Billy always amounted more than anyone at the end of the night. It even got that noticed that at one point other lads from the other estate used to come especially to play him, and what was a relaxing night with friends became a boozy brawl because they accused him of cheating. Mind you the thought did cross my mind but i had also seen him lose.

I waited until Billy had recovered his breath before saying, 'You know Billy, if you stood in a bucket of shit, you would come up smelling of roses'. Billy reached into his trouser pocket and pulled out an envelope, as we began to walk on. ' You could be right Mozzy, here read that it came in the post on Friday, i meant to show it you last night but i forgot.'

Inside the envelope was a letter from our local textile mill with the offer of an interview for a job. 'That's great news mate', my reply came with a hint of jealousy as i handed the envelope back. It wasn't that i didn't feel pleased for Billy because i did, it was the fact that we had both applied to the mill for a job and i hadn't received anything. There was only a month left before we finished school for ever, to begin our adult life in the rat race and my high hopes of a job had just come crashing down and with unemployment at a record high, life after school was looking bleak. Noticing the depressive tone in my voice and while rubbing his chin, Billy asked 'I take it you haven't heard?'. Shrugging my shoulders i tried to smile as i replied 'No mate, was it that obvious?' Then giving me a friendly punch on the arm Billy said 'Just a little. Oh come on Mozzy, lets go your house and see what's happening'.

Dad was in the garden as we arrived back. Wearing nothing on top only his string vest, he sat in his old deckchair, glass of beer in hand sunning himself. At his feet sat Linda my little sister with a bag of potatoes, pretending it was a baby, brushing the gathered up plastic wrapping at the top of the bag with her doll's hair brush. Both me and Billy couldn't help noticing Dads balding head beginning to resemble a beetroot where it had caught the sun.

'Oh your back then?' Dad remarked as we closed the garden gate, 'Oh and Billy too. Good well you can both watch Linda a minute while i nip upstairs.' While Dad was rising from his deckchair, Billy proudly announced 'I got a job interview.' Dad patted Billy's head, then looked my way saying 'Have you really lad, well done. See what happens when you try hard enough Morris, you want to take a leaf out of his book'. Then shook his head as he proceeded upstairs. Billy turned to me and whispered 'Sorry mate, I'm going to go, got things to do. Give us a knock in the morning on the way to school'.

As Billy disappeared into the distance i looked down at Linda, who by this time had managed to liberate some potatoes from captivity and was looking less of a sweet 4 year old little girl and more like a baby coal miner after a shift.

'That reminds me' i said tickling her on the nose 'Bath time and by the looks of you little one, your after me'.

'Is there any hot water, Dad?' i asked as he appeared and once again took residence in his deckchair. 'I think so, your mother normally takes care of things like that' he replied 'She won't be back for a while though, she's with your aunty Ethel. Uncle Jim was taken into hospital this morning early and it's not looking good, he's been bad for a while now poor sod. You having your bath now?' Passing Linda over to his Knee as i replied 'Yes, i am filthy.' Dad looked at me, laughed and said 'Take a clothes peg for your nose Morris. I've just been in.'.....

.....As i sat in my own world thinking back the bell sounded for end of visiting. It was then i noticed the vending cup on the bed side cabinet still full of what was now warm coffee and realised i hadn't noticed Mom's absence in fetching it.

You know Mom's right, i thought. The more i look at him the more he does look like my Grandad.

Reaching for my coffee, i noticed Dad open his eyes and as he focused on his surroundings, sounding surprised he asked 'Bloody hell how long have you two been here?' Mom stood kissed him on the cheek and replied 'About an hour, our Morris brought me.'

'Oh Morris do us a favor lad?' Dad lifted his old wrinkled hand in my direction 'Pull that little finger for me. I answered with a smile, 'Your joking Dad, you will stink the place out.' Suddenly a voice chirped up from the next bed 'You want to hear him on the bed pan, sounds like Glen Miller.'

CHAPTER TWO

That's Life

The weeks after Dad's admittance was hard going, both emotionally and tiresome and it had come at an awkward time, for me anyway.

Starting a job as a truck driver was my dream job, i had planned and trained for it and training had taken me months to complete. However having your father admitted to hospital 2 days into your first solo week, i could of done without and with it being National deliveries i was hardly home never mind anywhere else. The only day i seemed to be home was Sunday, that day it seemed was becoming such an important day in the weekly calender and once again like clockwork i was driving to hospital.

Mom was sat in tall comfy armchair as i arrived, head buried in a newspaper. Apparently the nurses had brought the chair for Dad so he could sit out of bed for a while but to no avail. Mom was making good use of it though.

'Any news?' i asked.

'Ulcers' replied Dad winking from the eye furthest away from Mom. This was a code between Dad and me. He always winked when he was hiding something from Mom, normally money he'd won on the horses but this time it meant, he would tell me later.

Suddenly the newspaper rustled and Mom's head appeared above. 'Oh Morris, i didn't hear you come in, how's work?', she said yawning. Leaning over to kiss her cheek i answered, 'It's fine Mom', it's just not giving me much time to come here.' Fumbling in her pocket she gave me a stern look, replying. 'Don't be silly, work is work and you can't be having time off just to come here, now who wants a coffee?'

As Mom left the room i turned to Dad whispering, 'Right what is it, what you hiding from Mom?' Suddenly Dad's face had a serious look about it as he gave my the news, 'They think it's stomach cancer lad but don't tell your Mom, not yet – let me find out how bad first.'

I had to look away as could feel my eyes starting to water. Wiping then dry with my jacket sleeve i managed to gain some composure and croak, 'Dad, don't you think the doctors will tell her!' The lump got bigger in my throat as Dad replied sharply 'No! They have been told to say nothing until i say they can do. For god sake!, stop your sniffling, your Mom is going to need you to be strong in the next couple of months and i can't be doing with all that shit.'

Suddenly Mom walked through the ward door. Passing me my coffee she couldn't help but notice my watering eyes, 'What's up with you?' she asked. I wiped my eyes again and replied, 'Nothing, just a speck of dust in my eye.' In an instant Mom was taking a tissue from her pocket and putting my head back, saying 'Let's have a look.'

Mom was quiet in the car on the journey home, i think the tiredness had begun to take it's toll and she must be worried about Dad. After all she's no spring chicken and these trips to the hospital and back must take it out of her.

I was quiet too, contemplating a few things. How Mom would be when she finds out? How Linda will take it when i tell her? That reminds me, I thought, i will have to telephone her tonight. Then there was my own family, i think after all this informing, it's going to be dinner, shower and bed for me, i thought to myself.

I turned the key in the lock and swung the door open, i could here the chattering. Dinner was already underway in the dining room and as i walked in looking around the little child faces, Dad looked back at me in every one. 'I can't wait for this day to be over' i said out loud, and later as i retired to bed tired and emotionally drained. It wasn't long after my head hit the pillow, I was in dreamland.....

….....'YOU BOY!' boomed the voice like a megaphone.

There is only one person with a voice like that, i thought as i turned to see my form teacher Mr Garner. 'Thought you could get away with not saying good bye Morris?' Mr Garner grabbed hold of my hand shaking it. 'No Sir' i replied nervously 'I forgot Sir, with the excitement of leaving Sir, sorry Sir.' After looking me up and down Mr Garner bent over and whispered, 'Do me a favour Morris will you!, If your lucky enough to get offered an interview for work, which i am sure you will. Tuck your shirt in lad!' I looked up at him and smiled 'I will do Sir.'

As i walked through the school gates for the last time i couldn't help feeling confused, sad even. Twelve month previous this day was full of happiness as it signaled the beginning of summer break. I had a summer holiday to look forward to and no school for weeks.

Today was different, there would be no summer holiday

this year. Even so, i thought i would feel happy, glad that i didn't have to do lessons i wasn't good at anymore like maths and history but instead there was a hint of sadness at what and whom i was leaving behind. School always seemed to be about friendships and learning together. If you didn't like a subject or didn't understand there was always another in the class like you. This new chapter in my life frightened me somewhat and as from tomorrow there was to be no more togetherness, i was on my own to fend for myself and if i didn't understand, i lost out. Simple as that.

I was so engrossed in my future it was a while before i noticed Susan walking at my side. 'Oh Susan!, i am so sorry, i was in my own world, how long have you been there?' Seeing i was embarrassed she quickly replied, 'Not long', i just thought you might want some company on the way home!, after all we do live in the same street'. I looked at Susan and smiled 'That would be nice'

It was no secret that i was fond of Susan, i liked her a lot. Billy said i had a crush on her, which i denied of course but he was right. She seemed different from other girls to me. Other girls i found irritating, annoying and silly but Susan i found to be more grown up and mature.

Good looking too with a smile that could melt any mans heart. We did go out on a date once, to the cinema. We had a great time until i asked her could we make it permanent, she refused, saying she wanted to concentrate on her education. I understood and we stayed friends but deep down, to say I was disappointed was an understatement.

We both took one last look at the school, as it faded into the distance. 'Well that's it Susan', we are off into the big wide world'. Susan just shrugged her shoulders as if it was just an every day occurrence, as we turned to walk on. I spent the next few minutes in quiet reflection of the day before Susan asked, 'You had any luck on the job front, Mozzy?' I shook my head in reply, 'No! Nothing.' Putting her arm in a link with mine, as if to comfort me, she said 'Never mind, something will turn up, i am going to miss that place.' I looked at Susan and sighed, 'Me too!, More than i thought i would do.'

Suddenly Susan kissed my cheek saying, 'I will miss you too Mozzy,' and my uncontrolled reply was instant 'You don't have to. Well lets face it Susan you know how i feel about you! and school is over now so why not?' I was trying not to sound desperate but it wasn't working and i don't know why but every time Susan came near me, especially on her own, i melted. This could probably be the last chance i got to ask her, i thought.

'It's not that i don't want to Mozzy or find you unattractive but to be honest i am going to college then hoping to go on to university, it wouldn't be fare to you or me if we did.' Clasping my arm tight, Susan explained more, 'Once i finish college who knows what university i may finish up at, if at all. But if i do and i have to move away i don't want to be hurting someone when i do so. I am sorry Mozzy but it's still no, not yet anyway.' That's it then, i thought, it's over. My school age crush was being left behind, where it started in the school yard and it hurt. Yet i couldn't begrudge her, she was right. Her maturity had shone through, making me feel special in a way, or perhaps she was just letting me down gently? Who knows, i thought as we turned the corner at the top of our street. Susan just looked at me and as we approached her garden gate she said, Don't look so glum Mozzy, glum doesn't suit you.' Taking one last look at her pretty face i replied 'I don't think i am ever going to get you, am i Susan?' Then walked away.

Mum was in the kitchen as i arrived home, supervising

the cooker. While Linda sat peacefully in her high-chair with an empty bowl, her face, forehead and hair covered in spaghetti hoops.

'Who's a big lad now' Mom stated kissing me on the cheek. 'Me, i suppose' replying quietly, and as i pulled out a chair from under the dining table I quipped, 'I can't make out whether Linda has eaten them hoops or bathed in them.' Mom looked over and on realising stressed, 'Oh my lord look at you!. There suppose to go in your mouth girl, not your eyes, hair and look at my floor. Well your going to have to stay like that until i finish dinner, lady.' Mom tapped Linda on the nose to get her attention, 'Your the second person i have seen all messy today.'

'Really?' i asked 'Who was the other?.

'Billy' she replied 'He looked a right mess, he was filthy. What ever they have him doing at that mill, doesn't look a good job. You'd think they would let him shower or wash before home; they refused to let the poor lad on the bus this afternoon!' I looked at Mom in wonderment and started emptying the contents of school bag into the waste bin. 'To be honest Mom i ain't seen him since he started work. I'll call round later and see how he's doing but it doesn't sound good. On seeing what i was doing and looking a bit confused Mom asked, 'What are you doing Morris?'

'Dumping the past and looking forward to the future.' I explained, 'Well i am not going to need it anymore and i will probably need a bag if i get a job.' Mom had a look of sadness on her face, saying 'I know but it just seems a bit drastic, a shame really. However this didn't last long as in her next breath she uttered, Talking about jobs, you will have to go and register soon.'

'Well let me take my uniform off first hey Mom.'

Mom gave me one her stern looks as she wafted my head with the dish cloth she'd just used to clean Linda, 'There's no need to get sarcastic and with remarks like that, perhaps you should try the stage; it's not going to be easy for you and to be honest Morris. As soon as they stop my money for you, we will need a wage coming in. Sorry Morris but That's life.' Straightening my hair I reassured her, 'I know Mom, i will go Monday first thing.'

It had begun to rain as i departed for Billy's house. I couldn't help but wonder about his job after what Mom had said. I thought he was the luckiest lad alive a few week previous, starting a job before you were suppose to leave school. I mean how good could it get? He was working and getting paid a wage instead of sitting in a class room full of people, just passing time to the inevitable day. He wouldn't have to go and register unemployed and looking for work.

It felt like an age before Billy's front door finally swung open and the large frame of his mother stood in the doorway.

'Hello Millie, is Billy around?' i asked politely. 'I'll get him Mozzy' she said as she turned, approached the foot of the stairs and with one enormous boom, shouted his name on top note. Then assured me 'He's coming' as she disappeared into the kitchen. Despite her size and vocal range Millie was a gentle giant, a lovely lady. So polite and as a house guest she couldn't do enough for you. 'Do you want this?, Do you want that?' she would ask, so much so that it would get irritating at times when your trying to have a conversation. However as some people in the past have found out, getting into an argument with her is the wrong thing to do, especially with that voice.

It wasn't long before Billy appeared on the stairway

'Hay Mozzy!, What brings you here?' As Billy started to descend the stairs I piped up, 'Oh, just come to see how you are and how your job is going.' and giving me a thumbs up sign he replied 'Oh it's fine, hey i saw your Mother today'. To which i just laughed and mentioned she'd told me all about the bus. 'Bloody bus driver' Billy complained. After an hour i decided to head back home, safe in the knowledge Billy was happy with work. Even though he didn't like the shift rota much which was 6am to 2pm then 2pm to 10pm the week following but he was happy. Well for now anyway........................

…...............................What the hell!, i thought as i woke.

My forehead, back and legs were dripping with sweat, i looked over to check the alarm clock, it was 04.45.

Good i thought as i lent over to disable the alarm set for 5am, trying not to wake the warm cuddly woman under the mound of duvet that lay next to me. I lightly kissed her head as i eased out of bed and headed for the shower, checking in on the children along the way and for once the cold floor against the soles of my bare feet was a welcoming feeling.

Soon after i was showered, refreshed, fully awake and heading out of the front door. It would be 5 days of traveling around the Country, sleeping in my cab before i could return to my family again and even though i would miss them dearly, my mind was only on one thing. DAD!.

CHAPTER THREE

A Bit Of Fruit & Nut

It had been a busy day again at work and as i closed the tailgate on my truck i could finally think about heading to the local truck stop for the night, for a well earned shower, meal and rest. I was ready for it to

Tonight was my last night out before returning to the yard, and home. Head office had already informed me of my next days duties which consisted of two separate load's to be picked up in Wales. One in Swansea and the other in Cardiff, both before noon. Then home back to the yard with them.

Before Noon!, i will be bloody well on my way back by then, i thought.

It had been a hard week to be away from home. Even though i kept in contact via mobile phone, news over Dad was taking it's time to come through and i had started to worry more and more as the week progressed. And i would be glad to get home so i could visit and see for myself.

The truck stop was busy with fellow trampers as we

were known in the trade, all heading for the same places and with night falling, finally after an hour waiting, i was able to shower and head for the diner. Where after feeling fully refreshed i returned to my cab to bed down for the night but not before i carried out my nightly ritual of phoning home.

'Hello!' As the phone answered my little Sons voice came down the line. 'Daddy!,Daddy!. Mummy!, it's Daddy!' he shouted still holding the phone to his mouth 'Mummy is coming Daddy and i have a new train Daddy.' In the back ground i could hear the noise of my Wife coming into the room as i replied, 'Have you that's good Robert' Then as the phone changed hands the conversation became more serious, 'Hi sweetheart any news?' In the back of my mind i was hoping there wasn't as my Wife's voice sounded down the phone. 'Hi hun, no not yet. Don't worry if i hear anything i will ring, what time are you home tomorrow?' Feeling relieved and excited to be coming home I replied, 'Late afternoon, i should imagine, it's been a hard lonely week.' I could hear Robert in the back ground and by her in conversation whispering on replying, she was having trouble keeping him and his train off the coffee table. 'I know sweetheart.

Hey Billy called today, he called to let you know about a mill being demolished and said you would know which one. I told him about your Dad, he said he would call and see him when your Dads back home.' If he comes back home?, i thought. 'Alright sweetheart, i will see you tomorrow, i can hear you've got your hands full.' After we had said our good bye's i sat and thought for a moment, well i suppose no news - is good news, i hope.

I turned off the cab light, climbed into my bunk and snuggled down. But as i lay trying to sleep i couldn't help thinking about that bloody mill........................

…..................................I glanced at my wristwatch it was 07.30am. As i walked on i could see the tall chimney of the mill poking through the morning fog, towering over it's surroundings.

Not far now, i thought as i swung my old school rucksack onto my shoulder which carried the contents of a very large food parcel, wrapped in yesterdays edition of the Daily Mirror. Embarrassed at the wrapping i did protest, however it fell on deaf ears. Dads answer 'Oh don't worry, it will give you something to read as your eating.'

Three month it had been since leaving school. Three month of interviews, application forms and generally getting nowhere. So it came as quite a surprise when i opened the letter from the mill with a job offer, especially so long after my application, which was the same time as Billy's and he'd been working there since a fortnight before school leaving date. To be honest i had forgotten all about it thinking any chance of employment there had gone and i was even contemplating signing up for the Army, if my luck didn't change.

I was to report to reception at 08.00am, give my name and ask for Christine, who apparently would be my chaperone for the day. Even though i had met Christine before at the interview, it hadn't been held here and as i approached the main gate, on hearing the noise of the machinery through the half open windows of this large four storey building. To a young teenage boy fresh from school i found the size and scale of the place daunting. Noticing the sign that pointed me to my destination i couldn't help but take a sneak look through a ground floor window as i passed, to which the sight of rows and rows of machinery clanging with what looked like hundreds of women darting back and forth didn't make me feel any easier.

The thought of working in a room full of women had never crossed my mind but it did now. I always got nervous and shy around women i didn't know, which always led me to doing something stupid and making a fool of myself. If i could of turned round and gone home there and then, i would of. However the thought of the expressions on Mom and Dads faces if i did made me continue on and through the reception door.

To my surprise the room was empty, just a few desks with neat piles of note paper on, a coffee machine in the corner, a table crowded with magazines and a row of chairs along one side of the room, with a notice above on the wall saying "Please Wait Here". I checked my letter. It's the right date, i thought but where is everyone.

Nervous and not sure what to do i took a seat next to the drinks machine and started flicking through one of the many magazines. It wasn't long before the only door in the room apart from the reception entrance door, opened and a young girl stepped in and headed for the coffee machine. 'Hello there, who are you waiting for?, she asked as she placed her money in the slot. 'Hi, i have a letter to report here'. Resting the magazine on my knee i reached for my inside jacket pocket 'i think her name is Christine.' The girl chuckled to herself as i passed her my letter 'I will tell her your here.' she said smiling. Thanking her i returned the magazine to the table. It was only then i noticed i had been sat clutching a "Woman's Own" magazine with a front cover headline of "Does Your Man Suffer From Erectile Problems?" No wonder she was chuckling, i thought.

Soon after Christine entered the room, she looked so different from the interview. Gone had the pinstripe trouser suit to be replaced with black tights, a short skirt and a thin blouse that left nothing to the imagination. 'Morning Morris'. Introducing herself with her high voice 'I won't be long sweetie, just got something to do. Now there's coffee in the machine but it doesn't take copper, the toilets are just through the office door to the left but don't use the lock on the Gents it sticks. Two hours a delivery driver was in there the other day before we heard him, Oh we had to laugh!' As she closed the door and disappeared i stood to check my change for the coffee machine, as Christine swung the office door open again. 'Quick question, is it Morris or Maurice as in the french guy.' I was confused for a moment, i had never been asked that question before. 'Morris as far as i know miss, sorry Christine. If it's easier you can call me Mozzy, people do, i don't mind.' Christine thought for a moment then replied, 'It's for your work records. So it has to be Morris for the office but otherwise i like Mozzy. Great idea.' As the door closed once more i began to think there was more to Christine than met the eye. Oh pleasant enough but with a hint of fruit and nut, the latter being the case but i wouldn't mind trying her fruity bits, i thought.

My first morning was mainly taken up with filling in forms and informing me of the health and safety rules, which to be honest went straight over my head. Some of the words in the pocket manual i was given i couldn't pronounce never mind understand, so when asked if i understood, i just nodded not wanting to look stupid. I would have been there all day otherwise. As lunch hour approached i was shown the whereabouts of the works canteen and left to my own devices but was expected back at reception at 13.00pm and 'No later!' ordered Christine.

Being my first day and feeling very nervous about sitting in a canteen full of women, i opted to find a bench and get out of the way for an hour, eating my newspaper lunch in private. I had already been briefed on the afternoons activities, i was to be issued with my boiler suit and work boots and taken on a tour of the mill, ending up in the department i was to work in. Which up to now Christine had failed to mention and my works card just described me as a operative.

I wasn't really looking forward to the tour part of the afternoon, having to walk into them large rooms full of women; Especially as a new face. On the plus side though, i would be able to have a nose at what Billy does, i thought.

It was 13.30pm when Christine finally arrived in reception from her lunch, so much for the order of 'No later' i thought to myself as she breezed in straightening her clothes whispering, 'Sorry about that i been out for a bit of lunch and got a bit behind'.

Apart from Christine's late arrival the afternoon started off quite smoothly. I had been issued with my boiler suit and boots and the tour was going well and i was quite impressed being in such a large mill how Christine knew so many people by first name. However the winding room was next and Christine had warned me that the women who worked in there had a bit of a reputation for taking the mick, especially out of young men and as we walked in the first thing i noticed was the heat of the room, it was boiling hot. 'The heat makes the cotton better to work with.' Christine explained as a lady looked my way and piped up, 'You want to come in here on the night shift, my love, you would see how hot it is then!' Feeling brave I asked in all innocence 'Why is it hotter at night?' Then another ladies voice shouted from behind 'Oh it's very hot' she pouting her lips as if to blow me a kiss 'You can't wear clothes, we all work in our bra and knickers. That's if you wear them.'

'Really?' as i answered they all fell about laughing.

It was then the penny dropped and i realised they got me. Christine looked at me trying not to laugh, 'Come on, they have had there fun.' she said as she ushered me out of the room.

It was on leaving the winding room with Christine walking in front with her back towards me, when i noticed she had removed her jacket. Probably due to the heat, I thought. However not only was she now minus a jacket but sometime during the day she had lost her bra too and the flimsy white blouse was revealing all. More so when she turned to explain the next item on my agenda, the sudden change in temperature was apparent, as her nipples on each large breast pointed out and as a boy of just turned 16 years with no physical sexual experience my eyes were firmly fixed on this wonderful sight. Thereafter for the remainder of my guided tour every conversation that followed with Christine, i found myself talking to her boobs with a bulge in the front of my trousers. Finally, although disappointed that my peep show was to end, we reached the department where i was to start my working life. The company garage as a apprentice mechanic. Life could not be better...................

................Beep, Beep, Beep sounded the 04.00am alarm on my phone.

'Another day another dollar' i said as i stretched the weariness from my bones. Climbing from my bunk in the cab i thought back to my dream and Christine. I wonder what she's doing now' i thought to myself. Probably retired, i should think.

CHAPTER FOUR

The Good Buddy

You can tell it's November, i thought as the first Christmas advert arrived on the television. It was 18 month now since Dad was first diagnosed with cancer of the stomach and a hard 18 month to, especially for Mom as he underwent his treatment.

Dad was in hospital for a while at first on strong pain relief while they blasted him with radiation to reduce the cancerous tumours. Only when the doctors were happy with Dad's fitness would they operate and surgically remove them and that would take another 12 week or so, and even then it was fifty, fifty, whether he would pull through. We was all well aware what could happen as the Consultant had made it perfectly clear before Dad signed to grant his permission. Explaining there had at that time been only four other patients in the country undergone this new treatment, two had died on the operating table and one of heart attack soon after. Leaving one remaining, who was undergoing the latter stage of the treatment. Chemotherapy or Chemo as Dad called it.

Finally after a while we got the dreaded phone call to say he'd been taken down for the operation. I was in Scotland at the time, 2 days in to a 5 day tramp and i wanted to come home. It took Mom to convince me to stay out as like she said 'There's nothing we can do, it's up to him now.' However i was upset at not having the chance to see him the night before, to say goodbye and be there for Mom if things did go wrong.

Dad proved me wrong though. After a few weeks where he was very ill after the operation, he started to slowly make progress. Week by week he improved until he was finally allowed to return home to recover and carry on to his next stage of treatment, Chemo. Six month ago he started his Chemotherapy and how that treatment makes you better, i can't understand. To see Dad with a line inserted into his chest to which he's to live with until they end his treatment is bad enough, but more upsetting is no body hair. Also he's quite ill after every dosage of chemotherapy, lasting about a fortnight, then just as he's recovering it's time for another. Anyone who visits has to be careful and if they are recovering from a cold or flu virus they are barred from the house, until it's fully passed. As due ue to the Chemotherapy Dads immune system is zero and even a slight cold virus could kill him.

That's when Mom came up with the idea of the hand held walking radio's to communicate with each other if Dad was upstairs in bed ill after his treatment. Now that does take me back...............................

...................I had been working at the garage for about six week and even though we were working at the same company, i had not seen sight or sound of Billy. I was lucky my shift pattern was fixed and more sociable, requiring me to work 07.30am until 16.30pm Monday to Friday. So on the odd evening i had managed to call round, he'd either been at work or out. Even our Saturday night's had come to halt. Mum suggested he may be seeing a girl from the mill but I couldn't agree, 'No Mom. Knowing Billy as i know him, he'd of been round here promoting the fact.', i assured her. So on leaving work one evening i decided to check in on Christine, to see if she could enlighten me to what shifts Billy was on that week. Fortunately for me Dizzy Christine was actually sane that afternoon and without any fuss informed me, 'Billy is doing 6am till 2pm this week.' Great, i thought as i walked to the bus stop and decided to call on the way home.

As i was waiting for the bus i heard a quiet female voice from behind. 'Is that Mozzy?' I turned to see Hilda, Susan's Mother 'Well don't you look grown up in your boiler suit.' I was determined not to ask the obvious question but inquisition got the better of me and suddenly i found myself blurting out 'How's Susan.' Hilda fumbled in her bag for her purse 'Oh she's fine, don't see much of her these days Mozzy, not since she started courting. He seems alright but you never know with these junior doctors.' Junior doctor!, i thought. Well that's me finished how could i compete with that in my boiler suit and the more Hilda spoke the more my heart sank.

I got off the bus dejected, all i could hear in my head was Susan's voice saying 'If i have to move away i don't want to hurt someone, when i do.' 'I was right', thinking back, 'She was letting me down gently, it's time to move on and this time i mean it.'

Arriving at Billy's with my head in another world, i was soon brought back to earth by the sound of crackling. It seemed to be coming from his open bedroom window. I pushed the door bell again and again, still no answer and in desperation and forgetting i was wearing my work boots, i kicked his front door, which only brought Mr Peterson his neighbor out to investigate.

'Sorry.' holding my hand up in apology 'Do you know if anyone's in?' Mr Peterson looked confused 'You can bloody tell he's in.' he barked, pointing into his house 'I can hear that radio from in there! Can you tell him to turn it down, I don't know where he's got that bloody thing from but it needs tuning in, tell him.' Mr Peterson, scratched his forehead then turned to return inside, 'My Trudy has never been the same since he got that thing, didn't come home till this morning. Wife was going mad.' I pressed the door bell again 'Who's that your Daughter?' Mr Peterson gave me a stern look 'Daughter!, it's my bloody pigeon.'

All at once the front door swung open, looking quickly to see who it was Billy shouted 'Hey Mozzy, quick follow me.' as he disappeared upstairs, leaving me to close the door behind me. The crackling noise started up again as i reached his bedroom door. 'Look at this.' Billy pointed 'Do you know what it is?', he started to fiddle with a dial. 'It looks like a car stereo to me mate' i said giving it a good look over. Billy laughed 'Since when has a car stereo had a microphone, you daft sod it's a CB.'

He then went into full detail of the in's and out's of Citizen Band radio and how you need a name or "Angle" as it's known in the CB world. 'You'll have to think of one Mozzy, if you want to use it,' he scratched his chin trying to think of a name. As i looked at him, i noticed the daylight fading through his window, 'Who said i want to, i am quite happy watching you, anyway i better get off soon.'

As i got up to leave, Billy patted me on the back saying, 'You will Mozzy, there are loads of chicks on this thing. In fact there's a big meeting next Friday at our local pub, there's a disco. Do you fancy it?' It didn't take me long to think about it 'You know what Billy, Why not!'

The following week was busy at work as the majority of the company cars were being renewed and needed servicing before returning to the lease hire company, all fifty of them. It was one after another and at one point in the garage, we had four ramps on the go trying to get through them all. 'Not enough hours in the bloody day' Terry the head mechanic complained. Needless to say the days flew by and Friday was soon upon me, the day of the CB club disco and i had everything planned. It would be home for a chilled few hours, then a long soak in the bath, put my glad rags on then out. Hoping to catch one of these fish Billy was on about in this CB dating sea.

He'd better be in, i thought as i stood in front of the mirror, combing my hair. Noticing Dad behind me I turned to him, 'How do I look?'. Not saying a word he just stood with his nose in the air, sniffing like a sniffer dog. 'Is that you I can smell, what the bloody hell have you got on?' I cupped my hands to my face to smell. It seemed fine to me, I thought as I looked at him. 'It's aftershave Dad.' He wafted his hand in front of his nose disapproval 'Where the hell have you got that shit from?', his wafting got stronger, 'Good god Morris, you smell like the inside of a tarts handbag.' I reached for the bottle and put it in his hand 'I think you'll find it's yours, the one Mom bought you for Christmas.' Dad looked at the bottle to inspect it, 'Well it doesn't smell like that on me.' As i grabbed my jacket off the clothes peg, he disappeared into the kitchen protesting to Mom. I had not even opened the front door when i heard her say 'What's wrong with it?, if it's good enough for Henry Cooper, it's good enough for you!'

On arriving at Billy's house i noticed he seemed a little stressed and by the amount of the empty beer can's on his bedside cabinet, he was well on the booze already. I pointed to the cabinet, 'I see you didn't save me one.' Billy looked at me confused 'Oh sorry mate, i've been having a right time tonight with this bloody thing and i forgot,' he pointed to the radio. To my eyes the Cb radio looked fine, all the power was there, the lights were all glowing 'Whats wrong with it,' i asked tapping the top of the casing. 'Nothing's wrong with it technically,,Mozzy. It's what i have done or may have done on it that's bugging me,' he passed me the can to take a drink, 'I think i got us date tonight.' he announced. I nearly choked as i tried to swallow, 'What!, Billy you've not?,' he sat with his head down and nodded. This annoyed me slightly, even though my mission that night was to try and meet someone, date them and hopefully gain sexual experience. Helping me to wash Susan out of my hair, i wanted to at least be able to choose them myself. I couldn't be angry with him though, as i know if Billy does something it's always with best intentions. 'So Billy, what do they look like?' He scratched his chin 'Not a clue Mozzy. i was just talking to them both on this last night, they seem alright. One's called arctic girl and the others called cats-eyes, before i knew it i was arranging to meet them at the pub tonight.'

As i lifted the can to my lips to take another drink a thought came into my mind, 'Billy, if you don't know what they look like, how will we know who they are in a crowd of people.' As we made our way to the door, he explained 'They'll be the ones in the sweat shirts.' Walking down his garden path, i gave Billy a friendly punch in his shoulder 'You know mate you were right about that bloody CB, it's like a take away and you even got us a date to order.' Realising I had warmed to the idea he smiled and joked 'Well, i am having number 69'.

The place was crowded as we arrived, bodies in every corner chatting away like old friends who had not seen each other for years. Feeling a bit uneasy like a knife in a spoon draw we headed for the bar, even though we were technically under age we both looked over 18 years , therefore confidence at the bar was not a problem and after being served we found a corner where we could stand, watching the door. 'I can't see them yet' Billy piped as he looked around. Thirty minutes went buy and there was still no sign of Arctic girl and Cats-eyes, 'Billy, i don't think they are coming. Let's go nearer the dance floor.' Billy looked at his watch, 'Give them another fifteen minutes then that's it, i can't understand it Mozzy they said they would be here.' Five minutes later the door swung open and to Billy's surprise but my relief, in walked our dates; Holding each others hands. Billy's eyes were as wide as dinner plates, 'MOZZY, THERE LESBIANS!,' he exclaimed. Picking up my beer i looked at Billy and pointed, 'Dance floor now!'.

Later, on the way home, feeling quite dejected Billy decided to vent his frustration on a stone lay in the road, kicking it against the edging, moaning, 'Tonight had been a right ball ache,' then fell over as he kicked another. As i helped him up from his drunken state, in the distance noticed a small gathering in front of a house, 'Billy, quick i think it's your house.' Running as fast as the alcohol would let us, we finally reached and barged through the crowd, finding Millie consoling neighbour Mr Peterson and as she stood with his small head resting on her large shoulder, stroking his hair she noticed our presence 'He's in a right state, Billy.' Millie pointed to her temple, 'I think he's come over all funny, mental like.' Then from the middle of the gathering came a voice 'Keeps hearing strange voices coming from his television, asking if he's there.' Suddenly Mr Peterson lifted his head 'I am not bloody mental, it's true I tell you. This is all since the wife had that bloody spiritualist here last Saturday. It's alright for her she's spending the week at her sisters.' Millie put his head back down, trying to reassure him 'There, there, don't get all fussed about it, she's back tomorrow, she'll get it sorted.' Billy just looked at his Mother 'That's a poltergeist Mum.' Billy in his drunken stupor then decided, explaining this paranormal activity to Mr Peterson, would be a good idea. However it was while i was lifting my eyes in disbelief at him scaring his neighbour half witless, i noticed the roof and the thin silhouette rising into the sky, from Mr Peterson's chimney stack. Stopping Billy in mid flow i pointed up to the roof 'I take it that aerial is yours?' He looked up, nodded then looked back at me, 'You bloody fool you've put it on the wrong stack and left the CB on, this week not only have you been having a conversation with the CB world but Mr Peterson has too.'..

....…....................It seems ironic, that now as a trucker a CB is just a very useful tool of my trade, I thought.

CHAPTER FIVE

First Passed The Post

Monday morning: However, unlike any other Monday it felt weird not having to wake to the sound of an alarm, yet the dawn was breaking and i was awake, a holiday week it seemed meant nothing to my body clock. Although as i lay back into my pillow, i was looking forward to enjoying the much needed rest. Spending some quality time with my family and spending some time with Dad, who was now in his fourth year in remission and today was his quarterly check up with his consultant. These days seemed special to him, like milestones in his future existence, so taking a day out of my holiday week to drive him there was the least i could do.

Even though Dad appreciated the free lift to hospital and back, he hated his children being present at these appointments, especially Linda who was now a nurse and understood the consultant more than any of us. Dad hated it when due to Linda's delving we found out the full extent of his operation, 'Oh you've got your own problems.' he'd say when asked. None of us, even Mom knew they had removed his full stomach until it was explained to Linda the reasoning behind his special diet of little but often. The weight poured off him and in four years, with the combination of Chemotherapy and this diet it's reduced his weight to 7 stone, less than half the man he used to be. However he was still here, I thought.

Later that day, arriving at my parents house i could hear the sound of barking and on opening the front door was greeted by a large dog,'You've got a greyhound!' Reaching for his overcoat Dad looked down and stroked it's head, ' Isn't she a cracker, Morris.' It had been a long time since i had seen a dog in my old family home, especially a greyhound and seeing his new pet took me back to when i was a child. One of Dad's hobbies then was training and running them and most of my childhood from the age of 8 to 13 years, i spent helping him with dogs. 'Hey! On your day off you can come and walk her for me.' I laughed and shook my head 'Oh no!, you can bugger off, them years are well and truly in the past now. Hey Dad do you remember our Shep.'.....................

.....................I looked at Shep. Dad was right, I

thought, he did look a cracker and large for a greyhound too. His coat was a golden colour with one distinctive black scar above his eye, where his mother had bit him as a pup. Although at the moment he looked more like a hippo on the end of this leash, 'Come out of that mud.' According to Dad Shep had the makings to be a good dog, very fast on the track and a great temperament, he should know, i thought being a trainer. A bloody good one as well, so his past had proved as most of his canine pupils had matured to be champions.

However Dad had grown disillusioned with the sport. It had become more about prize money and betting than a simple working mans hobby. He was beginning to spend more time training other peoples dogs than his own, as the owners would be paying Dad a fee for training and food, he therefore felt obliged. This all came to a head and stopped after a while due to one owner. 'A pompous little prick,' Dad called him before dragging him to his waiting driver, minus his dog. Later, i learned that the man had suggested, after his dog had dropped form due to age, that it be killed. That was it for Dad, one thing he did believe in was retired greyhounds enjoy their retirement as a pet and later gave the mans dog to Grandad to keep.

Before telling other owners to make new arrangements for their dogs, as from that day he was only training his own.

Therefore, Shep's arrival came as a bolt out of the blue. Apparently a trainer who was a good friend, contacted Dad to see if he wanted him free, as Shep had developed a weird problem. The problem being he'd started running wide all of a sudden, darting to the right as the traps opened and as the track ran in an anticlockwise direction when he'd been drawn in an inside trap, boxes 1, 2 or 3, he was running into other dogs to get where he wanted to be and staying on the outside until the finishing line. Mom couldn't understand Dad's reasoning, she stood there hands on hips, 'There's only you, who could want a dog who needs a navigator when it runs,' then threw a tea towel at him. Dad lifted the towel off his head and turned to Mom, 'Look! i know i can cure him and when i do he'll be a bloody good dog. At the moment he's coming 2nd or 3rd with this problem, on top tracks, so imagine what he'd do without it on local tracks. He'd be winning by about four yards, he's running further than the other dogs and still getting in the frame at the line.' Mom puffed her cheeks in disapproval then returned to her housework.

'Come on boy, let's get back home.' I gave a tug on his leash and we began to walk, after a short distance i noticed the large muscles on his hind quarters, 'Wow Shep, look at them.' Turning his head panting, Shep gave me a long stare and if looks could talk, that one would say 'Will you stop looking at my arse.'

Greg our new neighbour was in his garden as we arrived home, picking up the litter.'Hello Morris, is that your Dad's idea?' Pointing at Shep with his bright yellow marigold gloves. 'Oh, yes.' My eyes were fixed on his bright hands as he placed them on his hips. 'Thought as much, he's a good trainer is your Dad. I thought he'd given it up though?' As much as i tried, i couldn't stop looking at his gloves, 'So did we', i mumbled with laughter as i raced for the side gate. No wonder his Wife was well known for her bit on the sides and had gained a reputation, i thought. After washing Shep down with the hose, i let him in the house to dry and watched as he lay in front of the fire. Coming to the conclusion that he either knew how to switch on and off, or Mum was right to be concerned. The latter being the likely of the two, looking at the way he's spread out on that rug.

It was a fortnight later, as i sat watching Saturday morning television Dad popped his head round the living room door. 'Come on get your coat, you can come with me for a few hours,' Looking surprised i grabbed my jacket 'Where are we going?' As i put on my jacket Dad appeared on the front step with Shep, 'Bolton dog track, i got him a trial race.' Setting off in the car, Dad sounded really excited about Shep's race trial, however i did a very silly thing. I asked one question about the sport, to which Dad, thinking i was interested, treated me to an hours lecture on the subject and on approaching the track, i looked around to see Shep fast asleep on the back seat. He looked about as interested as i did.

The race trial's had already started as we arrived and the noise of the mechanical hare, whooshing around the track was prominent in the cold afternoon air. 'Morris you can supervise.' Dad made it sound such an important job but in reality it meant look after Shep and my first task as supervisor, would be to wake up and prize this future champion from the comfort of the car. However, Dad had appointed himself a less important role of talking to Charlie the race clerk about Shep's trail, 'It's important i speak to him Morris,' he pointed out. The fact Charlie just so happen to make the track bar is office was unfortunate. Charlie or slim as Dad nicknamed him was a good friend of the family and whenever we had a family party Charlie and his Wife would always get an invite.

Opening the door of the car Shep never moved, oblivious to what was going on, he lay curled up asleep on a blanket. 'Come on boy, you ain't going to impress anybody in there.' Nudging him gently he opened his eyes, lifted his head, yawned and lay back down. Well that's the sign of a real champion, i thought. Suddenly the whooshing noise from the hare started up again, Shep opened his eyes, rose up and jumped from the car. Ears pricked, he put both feet forward, stretched and sat by my feet looking up to me as if to say 'Well, do I have to walk myself there or what?' Quickly, i gathered his leash and gave a slight tug as a signal i was ready to move. Shep set off like a high speed train, pulling it's only carriage (Me) and no matter how hard i pulled at his leash, i couldn't halt his progress. Trying to dig my heels into the hard autumnal ground had no effect and he sped through the track entrance, pulling his trainee land skier behind him. As i felt my legs about to part a large hand appeared from behind and grabbed his leash, 'Whoa there, whoa boy whoa,' all of a sudden Shep stopped and stood still. 'Bloody hell Morris, what you doing with him?' Dad stood and stroked Shep's head to calm him as i looked on rather puzzled, 'But Dad,' i tried to explain. 'Never mind but Dad, you need to stop clowning about with him Morris, your going to hurt him carrying on like that.' EXCUSE ME, i thought as i dusted myself down, then still in a sulk followed Dad to the weighing room. Handing Shep over to the track official Dad turned to me 'You alright Morris?' Finally, i thought as i rubbed the strain on my inside leg, he does care. I'm second to the dog but he does care, ' Yeah fine.' We watched the official take Shep to a kennel to await his race then we went and stood in the near empty stand. 'Why is not busy Dad, i thought it would've been busier than this?' Dad straightened his cap 'It's only trial's Morris, these races are to determine if the dog is good enough for the track and if so at what group level. The time determines that lad but he's good enough, there's no doubt about that, i am just needing to see his problem.' Dad tapped the side of his nose. ' And let these buggers see it too, he won't have it for long but that's for me to know and hopefully these to find out.'

Charlie after speaking to Dad decided to put Shep in race trail number 6, as the other four dogs were proven open race dogs. They had been retired off the large well know City tracks and sold to owners who due to finances could only race at the lower league town tracks, so they were used to racing and would make the time needed. This was ideal for Dad as he didn't want Shep running with dogs known to this particular track, who were just having a training run, not today anyway.

As trail 5 got underway i could see a kennel handler begin to walk Shep down to the traps, in readiness for trail 6 and noticed he was wearing the red number 1 jacket. 'Oh no Dad, look!' I tugged his sleeve and pointed over to Shep, 'He's in trap 1, after what you said that's bad, isn't it?' Dad smiled 'Not really lad, i ain't expecting him to win but it does give me look at him properly, warts and all.' Trail 5 ended and according to Dad it was fast and as the times were being put up on the digital scoreboard, the kennel handler loaded Shep into his trap for trail 6 and as the final dog was loaded into his trap, the starting steward raised his flag for the hare to start. Seconds later the mechanical hare whooshed past, the traps opened and out came five canine bullets from their spring loaded gun. Shep ran straight for the first 20 yards then darted to the right, bumping into dog number 3 as he did so and as they reached the first bend Shep was last position. He was about 5 yard behind the leading dog as they rounded the bend then suddenly he picked up speed and as they rounded the last bend he was still out wide but in second position. Down the finishing straight he came, neck and neck with what once was the leader and as they crossed the line, Dad punched the air in delight. 'What a bloody cracker.' He lifted me high into his chest and hugged me tight, 'Oh Morris, what have we hear my lad. What have we hear.' As he lowered me down i noticed the scoreboard, first and second place had been given the same time, it was a dead heat.

Soon after, as we collected Shep from the kennels Dad was ecstatic, showing his pleasure by fussing Shep's doggy coat and kissing his nose. Shep however just seemed to take it all in his stride, not knowing what the fuss was about and as we left to make the journey home, i looked back and as before he was curled up asleep on the back seat of the car.

In the weeks that followed Dad tried everything to get Shep to run straight, he just couldn't put his finger on the cause of him darting to the right after starting. 'I don't know your a mystery.' he'd say after another idea to combat it had failed. Then one day Grandad arrived at the door. 'I've been thinking about this, he's been frightened by something,' Dad looked puzzled, 'What do you mean?' Making himself comfy in the armchair, Grandad took out his tobacco pipe and began to explain. 'I think in the past something has frightened him, his doggy brain has sub-consciously remembered it and it's become a habit.' Dad scratched his head and looked at Grandad, 'You might be right there Pap, the only thing is what to do.' Grandad blew out a large cloud of smoke from his pipe, 'Undo what has been done and i have an idea how.'

Early next morning after picking up Grandad, Shep's mystery psychiatric treatment began and as Dad pulled the car along side a canal tow path, i was still none the wiser. Soon however all became apparent when Dad set up his home made starting trap in the middle of the tow path, with the long grass verge to it's left and the cold watery canal to it's right. Grandad was 100 yards further down the path waving a pretend hare which happened to be a cut off sleeve of Mom's imitation fur coat. She'll go spare, i thought as Dad loaded Shep into the trap.

Looking up he waved to Grandad 'Ready, GO!' and pressing on the spring loaded lever the trap flew open. Shep, none the wiser raced out like a bullet and sure enough after 20 yards he darted right, only this time it was not into another race dog but a cold watery canal. Shocked initially but more surprised Shep swam to the edge where Dad lifted him out and quickly dried him off. 'Give him time to warm up and we go again,' Grandad nodded and soon enough the process was being repeated. Although this time on exiting, he ran as straight as an arrow. 'See I told you' Grandad shouted 'The old head wins again.'

From that day, it never happened again and Shep went on to be the best greyhound of my Dad's training career. Very rarely was he never first passed the post and on his retirement from the track , he carried on as he always did off track , as a house dog and friend..........................

…..........Arriving at the hospital Dad puffed his cheeks, 'Here we go again,' he moaned as i opened the car door to help him out and gazing down on his slender skeletal figure i couldn't help thinking. Yes Dad, unfortunately those days are well and truly over.

CHAPTER SIX

His Loss – My Gain

New years eve and as the church bells chimed midnight, we all raised a glass in celebration of the beginning of a new year. All except Dad, who was now fast asleep in his bed recovering from a long day and two small glasses of whiskey. An unfortunate disadvantage of not having a stomach was the effects of alcohol was rapid and multiplied compared to us lucky ones.

We were now entering his sixth year as a recovering cancer sufferer and according to his consultant Dad was a walking miracle, although at the moment seeing him tucked up in his bed you wouldn't think so. Even so according to my sister Linda, his consultant had admitted Dad hadn't been expected to survive more than 2 years after his operation, according to statistics. 'You know, your not suppose to be around anymore according to these figures.' he would say to Dad, i think that made him feel a bit special, really. Like a fighter. Over the last few month however, it was noticeable that fighting spirit had started to dwindle. His in take of food had lessened and his lack of interest in his hospital appointments was worrying. Arguing the fact he needn't go and they were just a waste of time, he refused point blank to go on the last one preferring instead to stay at home with Peggy his greyhound. 'I don't know, Dad. Happy new year,' i sighed as i kissed him on the forehead and left him blissfully sleeping, as i closed his bedroom door secretly i was dreading what this year may bring as i returned to the family gathering below.

As i walked into the room i was instantly kissed and congratulated on a new year by my children, niece and nephew, hugged and kissed by Linda and Mom then last but not least my Wife. Looking up at me she put her head on my chest and hugged me tight, 'How long have we been married, Mozzy?' i kissed the top of her head 'In this new year it will be 20 years in November.' She looked up and kissed my cheek, 'And how long have we been together?' i looked her in the eyes 'Oh, 25 years on and off, i think.' Then she smiled and kissed my lips, 'And when did we get together?' Putting my arms around her shoulders i held her close, 'It was new years eve, my darling. Happy anniversary.' How could i ever forget, i thought............

...............The air was cold as i made my way home from another hard day at work, with only a week to go until Christmas Day, the sharp icy wind cut into my face as it blew through my clothing and waiting for my bus, i watched the now familiar sight of festive lights twinkling upon Christmas trees carefully placed in windows and somehow this made me feel slightly warmer.

It wasn't a Christmas holiday i was looking forward to, however. It had been tainted by the announcement of redundancies at work and today i had received my notification, that i was one of the unfortunate few. Five years i had been at the garage, working hard and for what?, i asked myself. To be told by a managerial letter a week before Christmas, there is no need for my services beyond New Year was a kick in the teeth, the bastards, i thought. Then there were the friendships i had made along the way, good friends too. Little do they know this forthcoming works Christmas party, would actually be a farewell party for me and as the bus arrived i looked over at the enormous structure of the building; The building that once made me feel so nervous, years before.

Mom was in the kitchen as i arrived home, 'Evening Morris, your dinner is in the oven,' as she kissed me on the cheek i handed her my letter, 'It's not good news, Mom.' i explained and left it with her to digest, while i went for a shower before dinner. As i returned she was sat at the table, she looked up with a smile, opened the oven door and put my dinner in front of me as i sat. 'Never mind Morris, worse things happen at sea. Look at it this way, your now a fully qualified car mechanic and if you wanted to, you could work for yourself.' Then patted my shoulder to reassure me. Looking up at Mom, i realised, she was right, 'I never thought of it that way Mom, thanks that's made me feel a whole lot better.' Then feeling some what relieved i tucked into my dinner.

Later that evening a knock came at the door, 'I will get it,' Mom shouted from the hall way. 'Oh hello, come in, don't stand out in the cold.' she said before popping her head round the living room door, 'Morris. you've got a visitor.' Appearing in the dim light of the hallway was a tall figure, of which I had not seen for twelve months or more. 'Hey Billy, how are you?, come on let's go in the kitchen.' I had not seen Billy since he left the mill, he'd left due to the aggravation he'd been suffering from the women, over a girl he was courting from work. Apparently she'd pretended to be pregnant to which Billy denied, so they turned on him. The truth was outed eventually but it was to late, Billy had handed in his notice and left a month before and was now working in a garment factory. 'So what brings you her?' Handing him a coffee he sat at the table, 'What you doing New Years Eve? Mozzy,' i shook my head, 'Nothing and i ain't doing anything after either but i will tell you about that later, why?' Billy took a sip of his coffee, 'Do you fancy going to a party at the social club?, i bought two tickets for me and my now ex partner, so i thought it seemed a shame to waste them.' I just looked at him 'Not again Billy, you haven't gone and got in trouble at another works?' Billy looked and sighed 'No, she's dumped me this time, well and truly, for another bloke.' He's upset, I thought, now that says a lot for Billy, he must of liked her. 'Go, on then, i will come. How much do I owe you for the ticket.' Billy shook his head, 'Nothing mate, it's on me.'

Billy was surprised when i told him over my redundancy, he couldn't understand why they couldn't have left it until after New Year and told us then. 'How to spoil a families Christmas, there like bloody scrooge, miserable git's.' he said. Mind you he did bring me down to earth, pointing out that i was lucky really. As i didn't have a Wife and family who depended on my wage, unlike some folk who had received the same letter that day and as he left and the door closed behind him, i felt a lot better, no more was i feeling sorry for myself. Seeing him had done me some good, i thought.

My last week at the garage was terrible, after i had mentioned my news. It was full of people saying 'sorry' and 'how they couldn't believe it' then in the next breath 'They hoped i was still coming to the Christmas Party'. I just wanted the week to end and go home, bringing this chapter in my life to it's forced closure: and when it did, i closed it the way it began by walking the two miles home. As a stubborn two fingered gesture to the management world, that there not going to keep me down. As for the Christmas party, i didn't go. I couldn't stand there while Management wished me Merry Christmas and Happy New Year, these was the same people the week previous had instead of a Christmas card gave me my notice, i would've probably punched them on the nose after a few drinks.

Christmas day came and went, spent with the usual crowd, apart from Grandad who had sadly passed away 10 months previous and at 20 years old i still missed his stories. Grandma was finding it hard though, they had been together since the age of 18 and now being in her mid-seventies, she missed him so much.

However tonight is New Years Eve and as we both walk to the social club, for different reasons Billy and myself are determined to have a great night. The club wasn't busy as we arrived but as the night went on the room gradually started to fill and by 10pm it was standing room only. Rising from his chair Billy lifted his glass, 'Do you fancy another?,' i covered my pint glass with my palm 'No!, not yet mate, i am pacing myself.' Soon after Billy disappeared to the bar, I felt a tap on my shoulder and turned to see a young woman with long mousy hair looking down at me, 'Happy New Year Mozzy.' It took my a while to realise who it was, 'Susan!, is that you?' Gone had the school girl i once new, replaced by a beautiful young lady. 'Yes, it's me Mozzy, i didn't realise i had changed that much in five years,' i stood and kissed her on the cheek 'Merry Christmas Susan, you look great any changes are for the better, i can assure you. So are you home for Christmas?' Noticing Billy returning back from the bar, Susan whispered in my ear, 'I will tell you later,' then moving away, she pointed across the room, 'I am sat over there with family if you both want to join us.'

As i nodded my head in approval Billy arrived back to the table, 'Who's that stunner?', i just smiled 'Susan, from school.' Looking surprised he stood up and looked over to where she was sat, 'Bloody hell she's gorgeous, it's a shame she's with a doctor, which one's the doc anyway?.' I stood slightly to sneak a look 'I don't know Billy, she didn't say. Susan's invited us both over anyway, so we'll soon find out.' Billy picked up his pint glass took a drink then with one lifted high brow, he gave me a look of concern, 'Don't take this the wrong mate but do you think that's wise?, i mean, you felt a lot for Susan back in the day and you can't say it didn't hurt when he came on the scene, so i just think sitting there with her and him, well it might cut you a bit.' I put my hand on his shoulder as a sign of reassurance 'Thanks for your concern Billy but that was a long time ago, i have grown up since then. Let's face it.' I pointed to myself 'What can i offer her, look at her she's good looking, well educated. No Billy i have come to realise unfortunately, women like Susan only see me as a friend and nothing else and as a friend i am just glad she's happy.' Billy stood up, picked up his pint glass, 'Well, what are you waiting for Mozzy, we don't want them thinking we are ignorant, do we.'

As Susan introduced us to unfamiliar family members one thing became noticeable, there was no boyfriend present. 'I wonder where he is?' Billy whispered 'Perhaps he's working. Doctors do work New Years Eve.' i whispered back and as the night progressed, the more alcohol i consumed, the more i gained the courage to ask where he was.

'You alright Susan?' she looked at me and gave me a little smile, 'I could be better Mozzy but hey ho.' I was puzzled, that didn't sound good, i thought. 'I don't understand, Susan what do you mean?' It was then she sat back in her chair and told me everything.

How he'd been constantly cheating on her over the years, with other students at first. Then it moved on to staff after starting at a hospital. She always took him back though, somehow thinking it was her fault for not being a good bedroom partner. The icing on the cake was when she found him and a young trainee nurse together. She stopped at that point and her eyes began to water.

'Stop right there Susan.' I said as she wiped the tears from her cheek. 'Don;t you dare blame yourself for his inability to keep his prick in his trousers. Your a beautiful woman with a beautiful character and if anything you are to good for him. As for the bedroom, that's just his way of passing the buck because he knows, he is the one at fault not you.' I grabbed her hand and held it tight 'If ever you need to talk, you know where i am, i mean that.' Susan lent over and kissed my cheek 'Thank you, Mozzy. I will remember that.'

I looked at my watch, it was quarter to mid-night, 'What you drinking, Susan?' I asked as i rose to get my round in and as i stood at the bar i couldn't help but feel angry at the way she'd been treated.

The table was quite empty as i returned, they had all but one headed to the dance floor taking Billy with them. The only body left sitting was Susan 'So Susan, I take it your back at your Moms now then?' I asked as i distributed the drinks across the table in wait for the dancers return. Taking a sip of her vodka and coke she shook her head 'No, Mozzy, not yet. My uncle is over for the Christmas period and staying at Moms, so there was no room at the inn, so to speak. I am at the local hotel until Monday, then it's home to Moms.'

Suddenly the sound of the bell on church clock nearby could be heard ringing in the New Year and the crowd of people in the room turned into a frenzy of happy kisses, hand shakes and congratulations. I turned to Susan 'Happy New Year, Susan. Let's hope it's a better one.' and kissed her lips. What was supposed to be a quick congratulatory kiss, turned into a two minute passionate embrace. 'I am sorry,Susan. That's the last thing you need right now.' She put her finger on my lips 'Shssh. The only thing i need right now, is someone who cares and loves me for who i am.'

Later, after saying goodnight to Billy, Susan accepted my offer to walk her back to her hotel and as we walked it seemed like history repeating itself. 'We've been here before,' i quipped as she held my hand and as the outline of the hotel against the black sky grew larger with every step, the more i grew reluctant to let it go. Not wanting to leave her, just in case she had a change of heart.

'Well, here we are Susan.' The hotel reception was quiet and apart from the night porter sat behind the desk it was empty, and as we walked to the lift doors, Susan turned to me. 'Mozzy, do you want to come up for a coffee?' and fortunate for me, the rest is history.

..............It was 01.00am as we waved Mom goodbye

and set off in the car for home and it wasn't long before the children were cuddled up on the back seat, fast asleep. Apart from a slight coughing fit, Dad had spent most of his New Years Eve in bed. He'd never have done that years ago, i thought. Life and soul of the party, he was! and as i watched Susan lay her head back on the head rest, i couldn't help but think how much we loved each other and how much i was going to need her love when that inevitable moment came.

CHAPTER SEVEN

He Did It His Way

Suddenly my mobile phone began to vibrate against the table top upon which it lay and as the bare kitchen walls amplified it's tune, i carefully stepped down off the small step ladder i was using to decorate, wiping my sticky paste covered hands on my overalls, before drawing it closer to my eyes so i could focus on the screen spelling out the callers name.

'Hi Mom, how are you?' Putting the phone in the crease of my neck, i continued to towel dry my hands as the voice so familiar to me came down the line, 'Hi Morris, as fine as i can be. Are you going today?', i checked the time on the kitchen clock, 'Yes later this afternoon. In fact i was going to ring you to see if you wanted me to come and pick you up?' I could hear the relief in Mom's voice, 'Oh please, if you don't mind.' When will she learn, i thought, shaking my head. Looking through the kitchen window i could see Susan stood in the flower bed, pruning. 'Don't worry about flowers Mom, we've got some.'

It was raining as we arrived at the church yard and as

usual, Mom and Susan came prepared with an umbrella, meanwhile i toughed it out with a cap to keep my head dry. As we stood watching Susan arrange the flowers in the pot, i heard Mom give a heavy sigh. 'You know Morris, as much as i have tried, i can't cry,' placing my arms around her shoulders, i pulled her close to my side 'To be honest Mom, i think you did your crying years ago at the beginning, you were to busy nursing him after that to cry. So you just hardened to it, as you knew what was coming.' Mom just nodded her head in agreement.

After clearing away Susan stood back to look at her work. 'How's that look?' After nodding in approval Mom kissed her on the cheek, 'That's lovely, thank you. You wouldn't think it's been twelve month, would you! Eeeh this time last year Morris.'................

............The day had started like any other work day as a tramper, firing up the engine on my truck to get some heat into the cab and sorting through my paperwork for the day. Unfortunately for me i was London bound and not looking forward to the dreaded M25, the biggest car park in Europe as us trucker's call it and leaving my overnight stop at 04.00am, i was hoping to be at my first pick up in time to give Susan a good morning call before the school run.

With radio on giving me the latest traffic report, i was making good headway and at 06.30am pulled into my first destination, early. Pulling back the skirts on my trailer for the fork lift to gain access to load, i heard my phone ringing in the cab. Bloody hell that office is on the ball today, i thought reaching for my phone to see the name Susan.

'Hi Susan, what's up?' There was a short silence 'Mozzy, where are you darling?', this sounded serious, i thought, 'I'm just outside London Susan, at my first stop why what's up, is it one of the kids?' I could hear Susan sniffling, 'You need to get home love, i have been with your Mom all night, your Dad is bad.' Susan started to cry 'The doctor has been this morning early and he's not given him long, you need to get home, as soon as possible.' My heart sank 'Leave it with me Susan, i will ring you back soon, i am getting on to the office.'

Knowing it was urgent the head office relieved me of my duties and promised a relief driver would be with me within the hour. Also the car he came in, i was to use to drive home, fantastic i thought and sure enough he was.

On the long journey home it seemed like god was trying to put every obstacle in my way, from traffic hold ups to road works and for a while i thought i was never going to get home. Until eventually the traffic cleared and i had a free flowing motorway once more and after leaving London at 08.00am, i finally arrived at Mom's six hours later to be met by Susan with open arms and teary eyes. 'The doctor is with him, Mozzy. I will make you a coffee.'

It wasn't long after the Doctor appeared with Mom and Linda following behind 'This is my Son, Morris,' and as Mom introduced me i just asked him straight, 'How long and why's he gone down hill all of a sudden.' Rummaging in his bag for a prescription pad he looked up 'Well, i think it's his way of giving up Morris and saying he's had enough after they found another tumour in his intestine.' Looking perplexed i turned to Mom, 'I didn't know that!' Linda turned away as Mom looked and sighed, 'I didn't tell you because i didn't want you worrying at work, especially driving a big truck around. There was no point, he refused point blank any more chemotherapy and just stopped eating all together, i did it with best intentions Morris, believe me.' putting my arms around her i reassured her, 'It's fine Mom, i understand and i can't blame Dad either.'

In passing the doctor patted my shoulder 'I would say 48 hours at the very most, here get some of this from the chemist, it's a sedative to help him relax and go peacefully, there's nothing more I can do Son, I am sorry.'

Later that evening i took a break from sitting with Dad to run Susan home, collecting the children from her Mom's along the way, who'd kindly offered to have them while she sat with Mom and as we arrived home Susan lent over and kissed me 'Ring me if you need me tonight, if not ring me in the morning,' then after gathering the children waved as she closed the car doors.

Mom was stood in the hallway on my return, 'I have made up a bed on the couch as your old bed has long gone it's just an empty room now, Morris.' I put my hand on her shoulder 'That's fine Mom, i am going to sit with Dad for a while.'

Sitting in the armchair that had been placed in his bedroom so Mom could be comfortable on her nightly vigils, i stared at the small mound in the duvet that covered the shadow of a man, i had come to know and respect and love from being a child. He was quiet now, the sedative prescribed had taken hold.

Earlier, Dad had been restless before i arrived from London, hence the doctor. He'd been frantic, beating his chest to try and clear away the fluid that was forming on his lungs and making him breathless, causing his now skeletal frame to slide down the bed with every beat. It was a struggle for Mom lifting him back up, he'd grab hold of arm and look at her, as if he knew what was coming but he didn't want to let her go.

As i sat Mom popped her head around the bedroom door 'I will take over in a minute,' i looked closely at her dark tired eyes 'No Mom, you need some sleep, i will stay here for a while and if i feel tired i will sleep on this chair.' I kissed her forehead 'Go on the couch Mom.' and as i heard the click of the living room door i got myself comfortable and closed my eyes.

A few hours later i awoke to the sound of coughing and Dad beating his chest again, holding down his wild arms i quickly spooned the sedative into his mouth, as the bedroom door opened and Mom appeared, 'It's fine Mom, he's just restless again.' As i let loose my hold on his arms Dad lifted both hands to the ceiling above, like a child wanting to be lifted up by it's parents. Then settled once again, letting Mom and me return to our make shift beds.

It was daylight when Mom woke me tapping my arm, 'Morris, i think he's gone. I just came in to see if you wanted a coffee and looked over at him and i think, he's gone.' Realising what she was saying i stood at the side of the bed, Dad's eyes were open, yet his body looked asleep. I rushed into the bathroom and returned with a small hand mirror and offered it up to his slightly open mouth, it stayed clear and refused to mist. I closed his eyes and turned to Mom and held her tight in my arms. She knew then it was over and she was right.

Leaving Mom upstairs to say goodbye, i slipped out into the garden to get some fresh air. Leaning against the garden fence i realised i wasn't alone, Peggy his greyhound was at my side. My eyes filled and with tears rolling down my cheeks, she licked my hand to comfort me, as if she knew how i felt. Stroking her head i sobbed until a voice came from behind. Dads voice! 'You can pack that in,' I turned quickly to see nothing. I never heard it again.

Mom was on the phone as i returned from the garden, making arrangements as if on auto pilot, i suppose she'd had this day planned for years, i thought.

'I've rung Susan, she's coming down in a taxi. She didn't want you driving, you've got a good one there Morris.' I nodded my head in agreement, 'I know Mom.'...

...........As I pulled the car outside Moms gate and watched her open her house door, i couldn't help but feel sorry for her. She looked lonely without Dad, like one part of a double act was missing. Even so, Miss independence was just doing what she's always done and just got on with it. You couldn't put Mom down, i thought to myself and as we drove away Susan turned to me, 'I didn't know your Dad did the football pools. Your Mom said "He wanted to make you and Linda rich" but he never won.' I just smiled 'He didn't need to Susan, we were already rich in love and childhood memories, you can't beat that.'

God Bless You and Sleep Well Dad

DECLARATION

Information

The author of this work would like to express that even though this work is based on and around a true story, for identification purposes all names have been changed to protect certain characters within. Also this work has been published with the consent of all involved and even though most of this work is reality, some parts are fictionalised to enhance the script for the benefit of the reader, again with full consent.

The author of this work would also like to express that in the chapters concerning animals, i can absolutely confirm that no animal was injured, hurt or suffered duress in any way and was loved and cared for as a family pet.

COMMENT

To have someone who you love, whether it be a partner, close family member or close friend diagnosed with a terminal illness is a terrible life changing moment and not just for the patient but for all concerned.

To watch a person deal with this inevitable ending is not only heartbreaking but humbling as utmost in their thoughts are the people that surround them as they make their journey, to death. The word of description nobody likes to use due to it's meaning of loss of life and finality, yet we all take this one way journey from birth. Unfortunately, unless a person takes their own life, how we take this road is not determined by ourselves but by fate and sometimes fate can deal a terrible hand. Meaning some leave this life earlier than expected, leaving their loved ones to grieve their loss.

Grief for some comes suddenly and unexpected depending of the situation and sometimes as in the case of "Morris" our main character in this book, grief is made a touch easier by the expectation of death. Even so, whatever the case may be, grief effects people in different ways and people deal with it in different ways.

In writing this book the author was hoping to show from personal experience, how over time the hurt in the grieving process lessens slightly, to be replaced by happy wonderful memories of the person involved. Meaning their spirit, soul or whatever you believe it to be lives on inside of you and are still with you in some way.

Also the author would like hope any reader who is experiencing the above, by reading this work it has enabled them slightly to come to terms with their grief.

ABOUT THE AUTHOR

As a person, Marley West was born in the mid-sixties in Manchester, United Kingdom and brought up within a large working class family. A typical "Northern Lad" some might say, to which Marley is proud to be called and like many of his generation his working life began in the once industrial heartland of Manchester and still resides there to date, although now semi-retired.

As an author, Marley West uses his life experiences or "Northern Roots" as inspiration for characters and events in his work, hoping to bring reality with a touch of humour to the page. If you have found this work to your liking, please look out for more from Marley West in the near future.